Power Isotonics

Tension

Exercises

Power Isotonics

Tension Exercises

The Best Self Resistance Exercises to build muscle, increase strength, burn fat and sculpt the best body without the use of weights!

Based upon the Training System that created Charles Atlas

Power Isotonics was written to help you get closer to your physical potential when it comes to Real Muscle Sculpting Strengthening Exercises. The exercises and routines in this book is quite demanding, so consult your physician and have a physical exam taken prior to the start of this exercise program. Proceed with the suggested exercises and information at your own risk. The Publishers and author shall not be liable or responsible for any loss, injury, or damage allegedly arising from the information or suggestions in this book.

Power Isotonics Tension Exercises
Bodybuilding Course

By

Birch Tree Publishing
Published by Birch Tree Publishing

Birch Tree Publishing

Dedication

To all the 90 pound weaklings, this is for **YOU!**

Contents

The world's greatest workout method is now in the palms of your hands.

Charles Atlas have inspired more people to turn to exercise than anyone in history. In this book is the very same system Charles Atlas used to build himself into a powerful 180 pound muscular build and procured the title The World's Most Perfectly Developed Man.

The mainstay of the greats, Atlas, Liederman, and Macfadden, training systems are the very same exercises that are featured in this book (although Charles Atlas called them Dynamic Tension). They are Self Resistance Isotonic-bodybuilding exercises, this is where one muscle group resists the other to create muscle tension to increase muscle growth and strength.

These simple exercises can be quite taxing for even the strongest person. Charles Atlas practiced these exercises his entire life and this system requires no weights, no equipment and can be performed at any point, seated, standing, or lying in bed. These exercises can be done at any time and anywhere, which makes this training system perfect for creating and enhancing a powerful muscular body without weights.

Charles Atlas became a living trademark. Inspiring millions of young and not-so-young men, boys and girls around the world to be the very best they could be in life. Anyone can use these exercises to transform themselves just like the great Atlas, into a powerful muscular he-man with his method of Isotonic muscle-building exercises. This book is more than bodybuilding, this book is designed to enhance your overall health, strength and lifestyle. This book will show you first hand, by training you, motivating you, and teaching you how to build a magnetic personality.

You will increase your strength and gain confidence. Charles Atlas has inspired millions of young men around the world to be the best they can be. This book contains the most efficient muscle-building exercise strategies which means **YOU ARE YOUR OWN GYM!**

From the Publishers

Happy Training

Yours In Health and Strength

HOW TO BEGIN

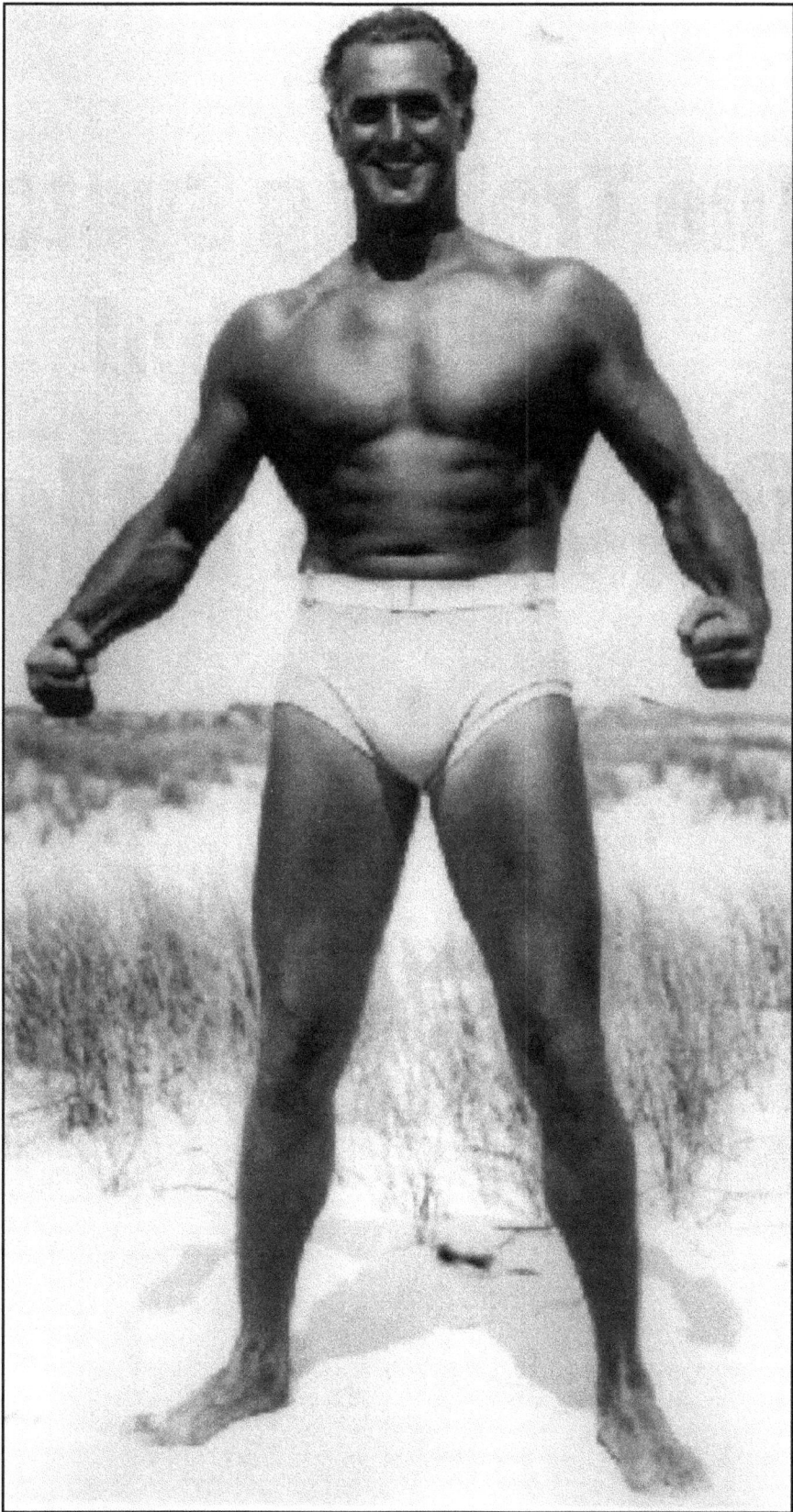

The Training System
that created
Charles Atlas

----

01   WHAT IS POWER ISOTONICS TENSION EXERCISES

Power Isotonics.

Power Isotonics are full range Dynamic Self-Resistance exercises that goes through the full range of motion, this is the mainstay of the Atlas training system.
One group of muscles supply resistance for another while going through a full range of motion.

Tension and Force.

How much tension should one use? When starting off use a light tension until you become comfortable with applying resistance. Practice using a scale between 1-10. Ten being the hardest form of resistance and one being the lightest. Use a resistance of 5-7. Far too much tension or force will create tendon issues, please use a light to medium resistance (force) this will increase muscle size and strength gains.

Frequency.

Tension exercises can be done on a daily basis. As much as twice or three times a day or more if you have the time. As stated above start off using relatively light to medium resistance that will allow you to complete 15-20 reps at a time before the muscle begins to tire. Or 10-30 reps depending on the exercise and feel. Once you have mastered the exercise movement you can vary the resistance used, but do not use extreme resistance.

---

02 CHEST EXERCISES

The truest SUCCESS is but the development of self.
Here is the first chapter, I am assuming that you value Health and Muscular Power sufficiently to be willing to pay for it in the full legitimate price of intelligent persistent labor. You cannot get results without effort on your part. If this is your decision you are invited to follow my self-resistance methods of development indicated in this and all succeeding chapters. To succeed in the building HEALTH and STRENGTH you must develop WANT POWER, resolutely making up your mind that you WILL follow the instructions no matter what sacrifices you are obliged to make.

You must be HOPEFUL, and expect the results assured that it will be ultimately yours. You must have COURAGE and fear nothing. You must have absolute CONFIDENCE in this System. You must have FAITH in yourself and these methods. Also, you must be PERSIS-TENT. Please remember that weak, spasmodic efforts will get you no-where. Henceforth, THINK Health. Make up your mind that radiant Health will be yours, knowing the results will be worth the effort involved. Throw off any tendency of negetive influences and keep the mind well occupied with thoughts of Health, Strength and Power.

As of today, you must curb your impulses, strengthen the good ones and positively reject those that are useless. The first great step is the reformation of habits. Where previously you would have directed your energies in certain channels that resulted in weakness you must now foster this new energy in methods that rapidly build up the body to glorious HEALTH and STRENGTH that will be yours forever. You are what you are because of your past daily habits. Today is a new day, make a change.

Let us build it up and not tear it down. Having signed up for this course, your object is to increase your HEALTH, STRENGTH and PERSONAL POWER. You must now conserve your energy for the acquisition of new and better health habits. Once they become fixed, you will experience no difficulty in retaining HEALTH and STRENGTH all throughout life.
To overcome your past injurious habits and develop better ones, you must bring your entire ATTENTION to the matter, you must think intently of the motives and the outcome involved and thus occupy your mind with better things, turning away from past habits toward freed

----

02 CHEST EXERCISES

REMEMBER, ALL EVIL HABITS MAY BE DESTROYED BY THE PERSON WHO REALLY DESIRES TO CONQUER THEM. Therefore, your desire for Health, Strength, Increased Personal Power and Physical Magnetism must from now on, be greater than your desire to continue on in your old way.

HERE ARE THE ELEMENTS OF SUCCESS IN ALL EXERCISES NOTE THEM CAREFULLY You can make your exercises a success or a miserable failure. You can make them monotonous and irksome, or you can make them a sheer delight. It depends entirely upon your own mental attitude. You should, and I want you to, regard all your bodily activities and exercises as a pleasure. You should look forward to them as a joy to perform.

The results will then be much more satisfactory and certain. Hold it in your mind's eye AT ALL TIMES your Ideal Perfect Physical Perfection. Think of yourself possessing the Perfect Body. You will realize that each time you are exercising you are getting closer to attaining your goal. Regard each day's exercise as a goal in itself. Follow the instructions faithfully EVERY day, and as you string these healthy days together you will have woven a healthier, happier, and extended life. Remember step by step and the thing is done!

In all your bodily activities put CONSCIOUS CONCENTRATED EFFORT INTO EACH MOVEMENT. Perform all your exercises with a WILL. FOCUS on increasing Strength into the muscle groups involved. THINK Power. THINK the muscles are growing larger, stronger, more powerful, while you are performing the exercises. Put energy into every movement. Focus on your exercises! Don't ever perform them in a half-hearted manner. Do not develop a lazy attitude.

Do not day dream while exercising. MAKE UP YOUR MIND NOW YOU ARE GOING TO PUT YOUR WHOLE HEART AND SOUL INTO EACH EXERCISE, AS GIVEN IN EVERY CHAPTER. UPON DOING THAT THE DESIRED RESULTS WILL BE YOURS. The first series of exercises will consist of those for building a solid foundation for the entire body. This chapter will give special methods for developing a strong powerful chest and acquiring powerful lung power. THE EXERCISES ARE TO BE FAITHFULLY PRACTICED EVERY MORNING IMMEDIATELY ON ARISING AND BEFORE RETIRING.

----

02 CHEST EXERCISES

This system consists chiefly of various exercises which aid in the elimination of toxins in the blood, at the same time building up the tissues, rounding them out, giving them muscular power and strength. Part of the secret of Health and Longevity of life lies in getting rid of poisonous, dead, worn-out cellular tissues, which if allowed to remain would prevent the perfect functioning of the various organs. One of the methods by which this dead matter may be eliminated is by properly directed muscular exercises, which you will be doing. You will understand these chapters better if you will read them out loud to yourself in a private room where you will not be disturbed.

The very first essential thing to do in securing radiant HEALTH and physical STRENGTH is DEEP BREATHING OF PURE AIR. We can live without food for many weeks, without water for many days, but we can not live without air for more than a few minutes. Air is equally a food as fruits and vegetables. As it enters into the composition of the body, its value cannot be over emphasized. Yet because it is readily available we ignore its real value. The first step required is to practice daily, FULL, DEEP BREATHING.

There are some teachers who advocate blowing out the upper chest to an enormous extent, but this is both useless and injurious because as you get older you neglect the deep breathing with the result that the cavities of the lungs are unused and this forms a suitable culture medium for lung problems.
What is advocated here is formal deep breathing so that ALL parts of the lungs are filled to it's utmost proportion to the size of the body without straining. The air you breathe must be PURE.

There are several reasons why you need to practice this deep breathing daily.
The air when pure is composed principally of nitrogen and oxygen. Oxygen is LIFE! The more oxygen you breathe the more health and strength you will get.
This life-giving oxygen furnishes the power to pump the blood through the heart.

02 CHEST EXERCISES

It assists in carrying off the waste products from the myriad of tiny cells in the body, and help to build new and stronger cells. Furthermore, it furnishes warmth to the body. As a result of continued deep breathing the lungs are developed, the chest expands, the ribs are thrown upward and outward, flat chest is overcome, and the deep breather is likely to be forever free from the symptoms of chest and lung problems.

Do not be afraid to breathe deeply and fully at all times, especially when outdoors when away from crowds. Do not be afraid of night air. Although the night air is not laden with the sun's healthful rays, it is often purer than the air we breathe during the day, because all the accumulated dust, dirt and smoke has had a chance to settle. There is no need to be afraid of mild drafts for a draft is simply air in motion, and contrary to the popular belief it is really beneficial. You should learn to welcome these cooling drafts of pure, vitalizing air as health builders.

Of course a strong draft is not desirable. Practice this deep, full breathing every morning and night! Self-resistance is the secret non-apparatus method - the same method that built Charles Atlas and millions of pupils throuthout the world. Remember - Self-resistance methods can help you, but only if you are willing to follow the instructions carefully. PROPER POSTURE, one of the first requirements in developing a MAGNETIC PERSONALITY is the assuming of a proper bodily posture while standing, walking and sitting. Nothing indicates a REAL MAN more than the way in which he holds himself.

If your chest is sunken and your stomach sticking out, you cannot stand out as a man with PERSONALITY. You are especially urged to concentrate on this and make sure that you hold yourself upright, walk with dignity and keep your chin up. HOLD YOUR SPINE ERECT. PUT YOUR SHOULDERS FIRMLY BACK. Make them square. HOLD your abdomen in without forcing. Breathe deeply and naturally, walk properly plus, avoid a slouching attitude. While sitting keep your body erect, keep your feet under your seat, and refrain from flopping down in a lazy fashion. LOOK ALIVE AT ALL TIMES. In this way you FEEL self-confident and successful.

----

02 CHEST EXERCISES

You will be able to take the world by storm. You WILL be successful. At various intervals during the day stretch upwards with the hands above the head. Endeavor to reach the ceiling a dozen times a day. This will increase your flexibility, loosen up the vertebrae of the spinal colume. Perform this movement daily and it will become a habit. This will increase your self confidence, plus aid in maintaining proper posture.

In fact, by assuming a correct posture while sitting and standing, you help overcome constipation, prevent rupture, fill the lungs with air, and improve every vital organ. This is accomplished by the muscles and internal viscera having an opportunity to expand and allow the free, normal passage of blood to all parts of the body, which is hindered when the abdominal region is relaxed and protruding.

Bear in mind at all times correct posture for Health, Strength and Personality. HERE ARE THE SPECIAL EXERCISES FOR DEVELOPING A POWERFUL CHEST Artists, Doctors, Scientists, Sculptors and Physical Culture Experts have declared that Charles Atlas had the largest and most perfectly developed pectoral (chest) muscles of anyone they have ever seen.

The tremendous strength of Charles Atlas's enormous shoulders and powerful arms is due to his muscular chest development. Atlas's chest measured 47 inches normal - not expanded, ten or twelve inches more than the average individual's. Do not despair! Charles Atlas was once known as flat chested. Charles Atlas came to realize the importance of a great POWERFUL chest played in search for robust health.

Today no-one wants a flat, sunken chest. You should strive diligently to possess a powerful, muscular chest for two important reasons. Firstly, because it gives unusual strength just like the abdominal wall to the entire body, and secondly, because it adds contour and symmetrical development, giving grace, poise and self confidence.

02 CHEST EXERCISES

A full round chest is an indication of strength, vitality and never-ending energy. It insures a strong healthy pair of lungs; a powerful heart, and the promise of an extended life. MASTER METHODS FOR ACQUIRING GREAT INTERNAL STRENGTH.

These unique and very effective methods are used for acquiring great internal strength and building up your chest and every muscle in your body. Follow these instructions faithfully DAY BY DAY, perform them all with CONSCIOUS effort, concentrating earnestly on what you do, and you will be more than delighted with the results. Now for the splendid special exercises, which can give you a MASSIVE and POWERFUL chest.

Be sure to take these special movements regularly EVERY DAYwithout fail. Perform these, and all other movements, where possible, in front of a large mirror, with your shirt off. The secret of acquiring an enormous, ripped chest is persistence of the dipping exercise, which should be performed DAILY.

02 CHEST EXERCISES

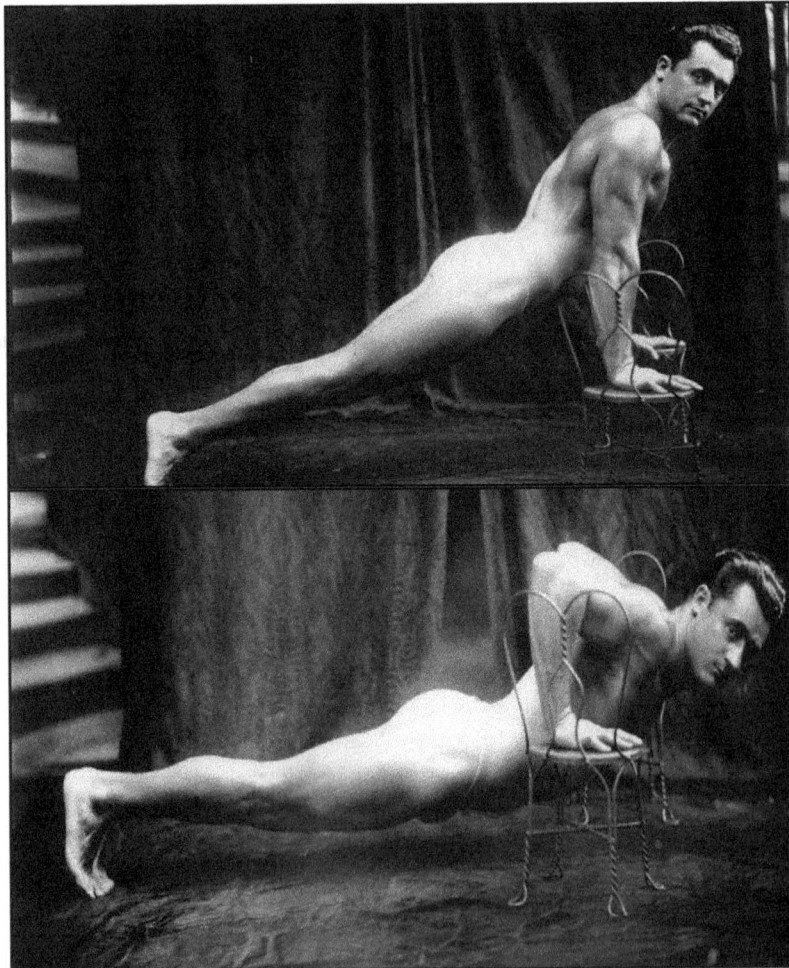

Incline Pushups

This exercise is the Granddaddy of all upper-body exercises. This was his key upper-body exercise for the chest. It's the best upper-body builder. This exercise is performed exactly as shown. Place your hands on two chairs that are 15 inches high, the higher you go the greater pre-stretch there is. At the bottom position to enhance muscle-building stimuli pause at the bottom for 2 seconds before reversing the movement. Perform 15-25 reps per set.

02 CHEST EXERCISES

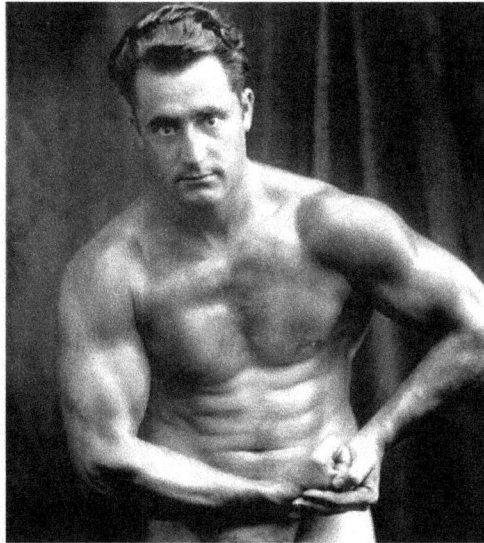

Across the body chest press

Here is an excellent exercise for the chest. Place your right fist in your left hand at the level of you right hip elbows bent. Against resistance of the left arm press the right arm towards the left hip resisting with the left hand. Perform 3 sets at 15-20 reps.

02 CHEST EXERCISES

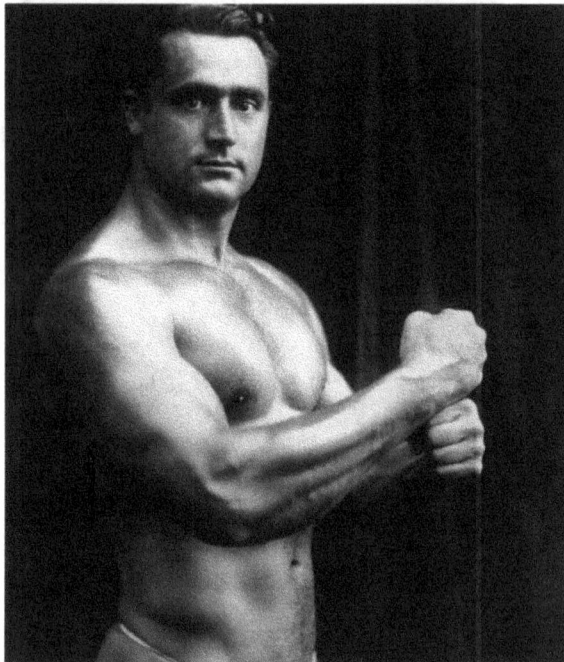

Stiff Arm Pulldown

Begin with your hands placed level with your shoulders right hand over left. Startpushing with the right arm downwards while resisting with the left arm. While maintaining tension, lower the tension with the bottom arm just enough to allow movement of a full range of motion towards the thighs then reverse the direction by pushing up with the bottom hand while resisting with the top arm. Continue for 15-20 reps at 3 sets.

----

02 CHEST EXERCISES

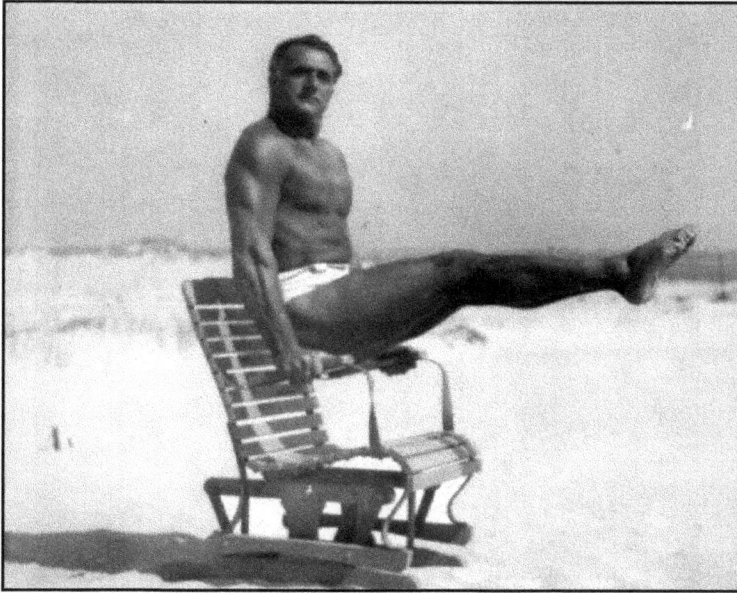

Chest chair dips

In the position shown raise the body up and down as many times as you can in sets of 15-20 reps. This dipping stimulates the lower chest muscles to its maximum.

02 **CHEST EXERCISES**

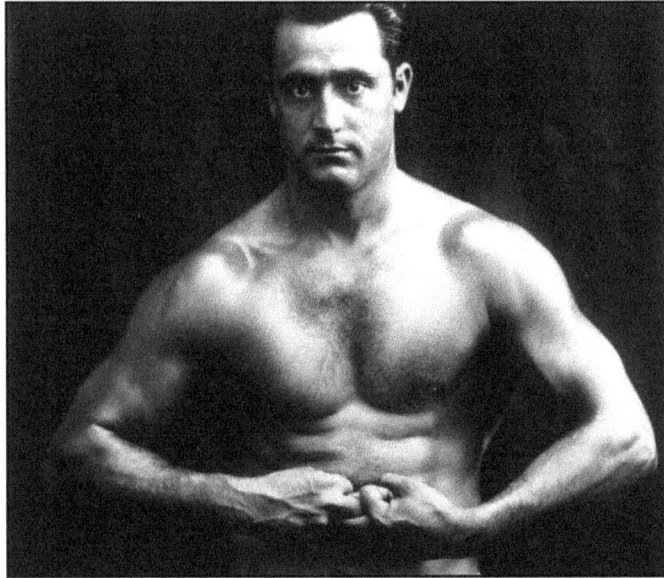

Up and over dynamic Isometric pull

Grip the middle of each hand as shown. Pull outwards powerfully while raising the arms overhead, then behind the head. Maintaining the tension of the pull, then reverse the position while maintaining the tension back at the start position shown. Perform 3 sets of 20 reps per set.

---

03 SHOULDER EXERCISES

Whenever I think of the shoulders I associate them with massiveness and great strength. I use the expressive term - broad powerful shoulders - as an indication of one of the dominating parts of the body. However, few of us have shoulders that we are proud of! The exercises fully described within this chapter will soon give you a coat of muscles of unusual POWER.

You must put energy and strong resistance into all the motions, performing them with diligence and regularity. With continued daily practice it is surprising how quickly you will note the remarkable increase in size and power the shoulders will develop. Let nothing discourage you from doing all you can to make your shoulders massive.

There are several exercises you can perform that will increase the development of the shoulders, such as the dipping exercises given at the beginning of this book will supply considerable exercise to the shoulders. If you would be successful in business you must be industrious; likewise in your exercises. It requires unwavering attention, great concentration and will-power to persistently continue these movements, stay focused and you will be successful.

03 SHOULDER EXERCISES

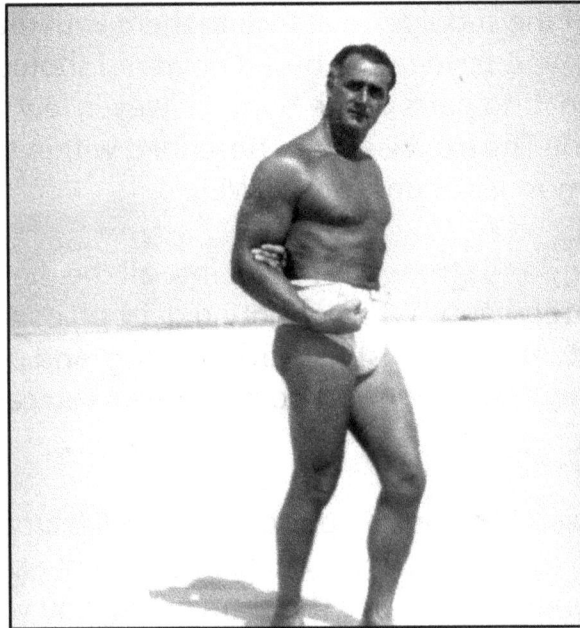

Isometric Forward press

This is an isometric motion meaning (no isotonic-full-range movement takes place). Go into the position as shown, allow your arm to go slightly backwards now press the arm forward as you resist with the left arm. The arm will come forward for a few inches, but the key is to hold it. Hold for a count of 20-30 seconds at 3 sets each arm. **PLEASE DO NOT HOLD YOUR BREATH!**

03 SHOULDER EXERCISES

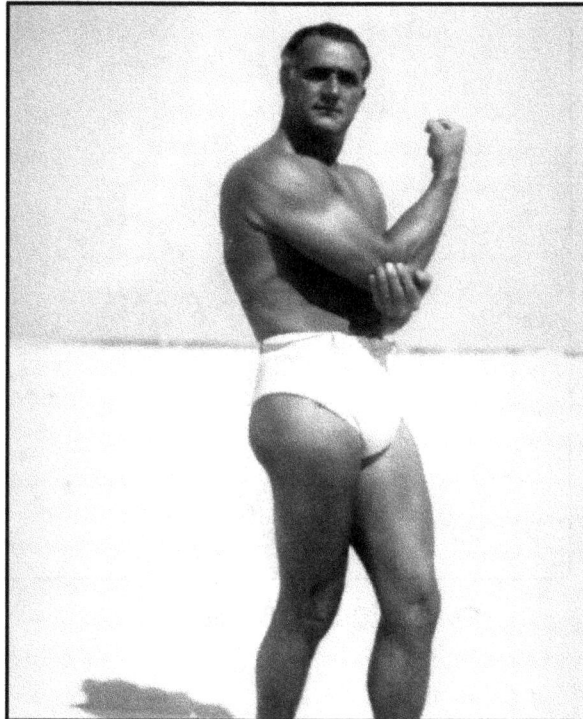

Across the body pulls

Bring the right elbow across the chest and grasp the left elbow with a firm grip. Slowly force the right elbow across the body towards the right hip resisting with the left hand. This exercise adds strength and development to the rear shoulder muscles and upper back. Perform 3 sets of 15-20 reps.

03 SHOULDER EXERCISES

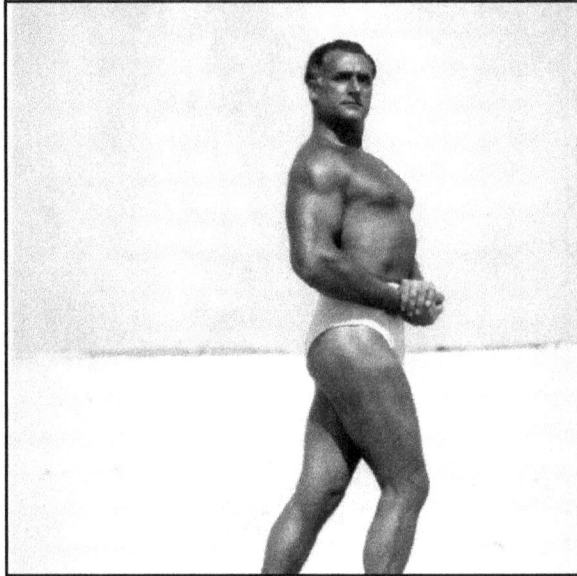

Side lateral raises

Grasp the right arm that is at your side as in the picture. Now raise the arm outwards towards the side contracted position resisting with the right arm. Perform 15 reps then switch arms, 3 sets each side.

----

04 NECK EXERCISES

We will now look at some self-resistance type movements for strengthening the upper Spine and Muscles of the upper traps. IMPORTANT! The first movement of all these exercises are to be performed with all parts entirely relaxed so that all the muscles are thoroughly pre-stretched. In the second movement, it is important that you stretch the muscles involved to the full range of motion.
This pre-stretched state is of special value in increasing hormonal release.

SPECIAL EXERCISES

The kidneys are glandular organs and their strength is of prime importance and must be maintained at all times. They are part of the body's vital organs, and as such demand special attention and care. While they are deep-seated there is a number of potent exercises which are frequently found useful in strengthening these small but necessary organs.

EXERCISES FOR THE NECK

It seems unnecessary to mention the importance the neck plays in the general scheme of physical perfection. The ox has a tremendous neck-while the animal is tugging at a heavy load, but this cannot compare with the lion whose neck is longer, more supple and slender, capable of immense power. This is the kind you wish to possess. The special exercises in this course will give you a neck with great strength and power, but you must practice each exercise diligently.

You cannot get a powerful neck on a massive pair of shoulders by merely dreaming of it. You have to DO your exercises EACH DAY, every day, until you have a strong, powerful neck muscles. While some of these exercises are very simple they are nevertheless very effective; you can, however, apply light tension at first.

----

04 NECK EXERCISES

EXERCISES FOR THE FACE

The facial muscles can become strong again with some daily tense and squeeze exercises. Flabby cheeks will become stronger and firmer, wrinkles eliminated, double chin will disappear- by effective facial exercises. Hollow cheeks are the hardest to overcome. Indeed it is practically impossible with some faces, especially where the upper cheek bones are very prominent. Often people with large cheek bones have quite round faces, but they appear somewhat hollow owing to the protruding bones.

Now lets look at some exercises for the face, Close mouth tightly and blow out the face as full as possible, and push the tongue into the right cheek and then into the left. Open the mouth wide as in yawning and stretch it open still wider.
Screw the face up on one side and stretch the other side. Do this alternately.
Get hold of the cheeks with the hands and pull them outwards and relax.

Gently massage the face with the hand by pressing the flesh from the nose out-wards to the ears. Bathe the face occasionally with very hot water and finish off with cold wet cloths. This freshens the face and gives a rich ruddy glow of radiant health. After this, pull the face into all manner of contortions, remembering exercise always helps toward perfection. It reduces fat cheeks and builds up hollow ones. Give the face the careful consideration it deserves.

04 NECK EXERCISES

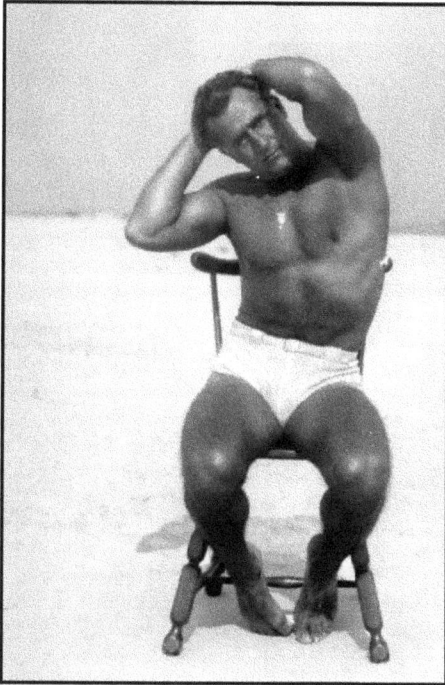

Side to side neck press

Bend your head as close as you can to the shoulder as shown. Place the left hand on the left side of the head and press the head to the opposite shoulder while resisting with the hand. Followed by placing the right hand on the right side and press the head back to the starting position as before. Dual action left then right. Remember use a light tension and once the neck becomes more conditioned and stronger increase the tension.

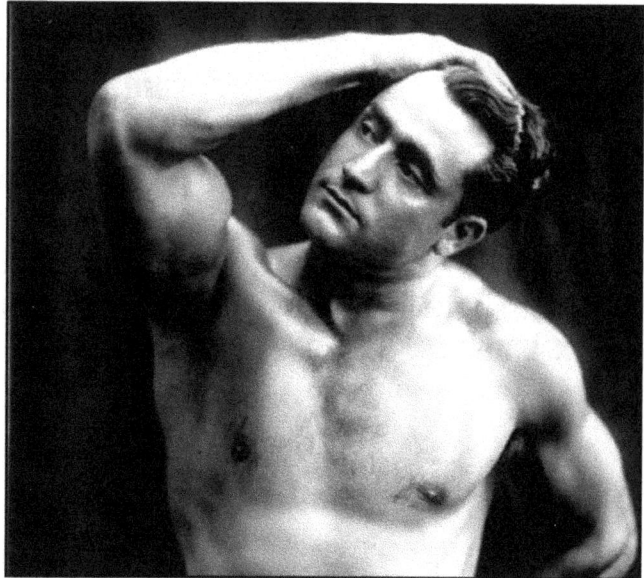

04 NECK EXERCISES

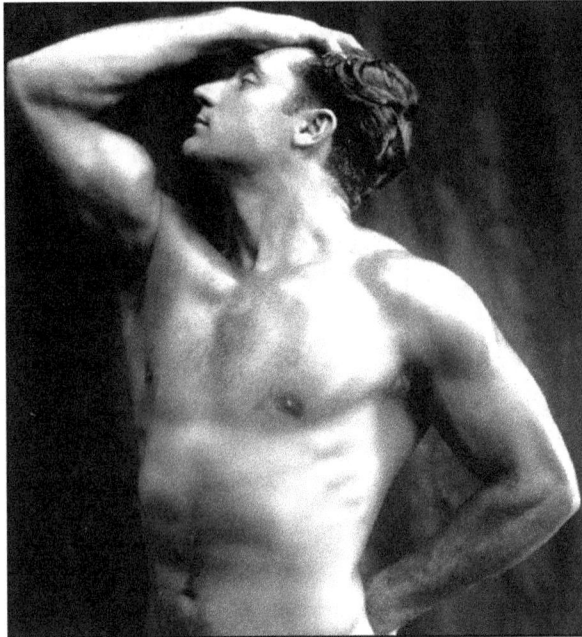

Forward Neck Press

With your head tilted back place your hand on your forehead. Now slowly press your head forward and resist the movement slightly with light tension towards your upper chest. Always use a light tension to the neck.
As your strength increases use a little more force but not too much tension.
Breathe Normal.

04 KIDNEY EXERCISES

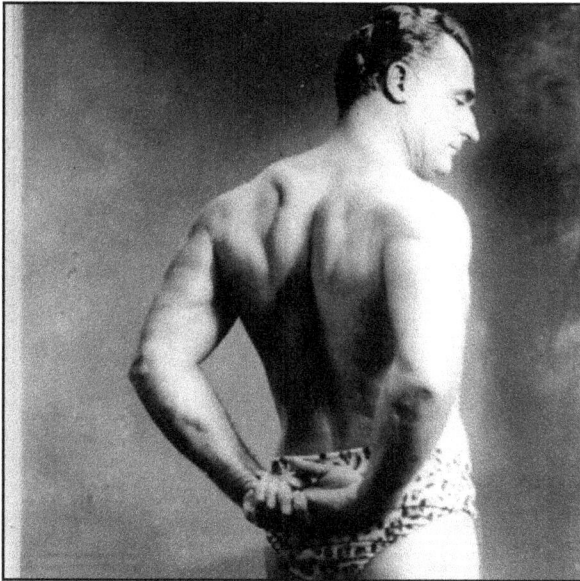

(Kidneys)

Grasp hands as pictured and turn to the left then as far to the right as possible. Continue in the fashion each side for 20 reps each.

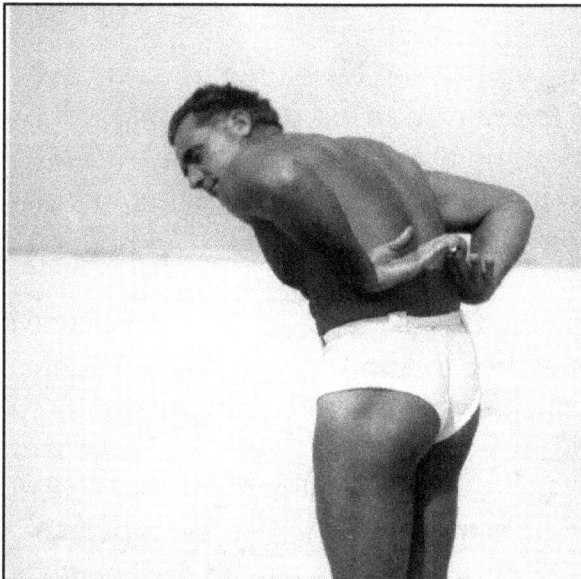

(Kidneys)

With the edges of your hands, chop the entire region of theback, as far as you can reach. A powerful but natural stimulant to liver and kidneys.

---

05   UPPER BACK EXERCISES

Everyone loves a strong, powerful back. It seems to be synonymous with tremendous power. The many layers of muscles on the back are quickly developed by self-resistance exercises, which should encourage you to perform each exercise in this series faithfully and intelligently.

It is not necessary to go into minute details, giving you the names of all the various muscles in this region, but if you will persistently go through the movements here suggested you will speedily acquire powerful, muscular back, with power packed endless power along the spinal erectors as well. Please perform all the exercises each morning and evening.

Make up your mind that each day you will spend at least half an hour in the morning and half an hour in the evening REGARDLESS- building a muscular body, increasing your strength and power throughout your body. We both know, it's worth it! Increasing your health and strength is more valuable to you than anything else. For without health and strength you are DONE.

Forget about making up excuses stating you do not have time. You do have twenty-four hours each and every day the same as everyone else. Make time to keep your body healthy and in fantastic condition, you need to. This SYSTEM is giving you the very best self-resistance methods for quickly adding muscular power and strength to enhance your present physique.

Be faithful to yourself by carefully following these directions and you will be more than satisfied with your bargain. Muscles, health and strength will not come by merely wishing for them. You have to buckle down and work for increasing the size of those muscles. However, the results from the efforts you make will amaze you, your family and friends. Perform every exercise as directed until you feel a good pump within the muscles. Always remember it's the last few reps that make the increase, and give you the increased tension you are aiming for. Focus on these words, PRACTICE, PERSEVERANCE and PATIENCE WIN - ALWAYS.

----

05   UPPER-BACK EXERCISES

Become a winner- a winner of strength gains and muscle size. Keep practicing, persevere at all costs, and be patient. Now it is very necessary to put enough effort into each and every exercise, but I earnestly request you NOT to apply too much tension or strain. Here is an infallible method to determine when you have performed an exercise a sufficient number of times. It is to continue UNTIL THE MUSCLES ARE SERIOUSLY PUMPED UP AND BURNING.

A very effect way of loosening up the tissues, bring fresh blood and oxygen to the muscles involved is to massage and stretch the muscles being worked, this removes poisonous waste matter, prevents muscle soreness after exercise. Now let us look at some muscle-building exercises.

---

05 UPPER-BACK EXERCISES

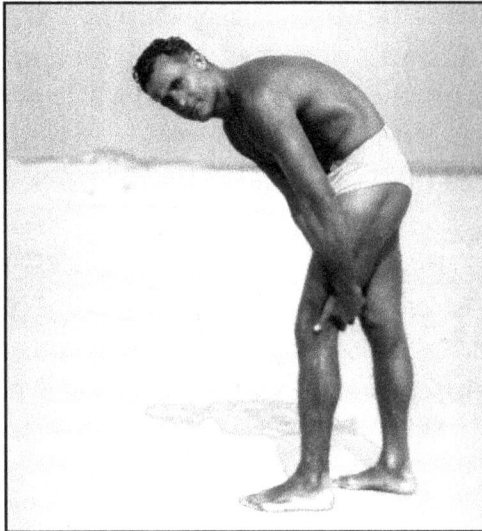

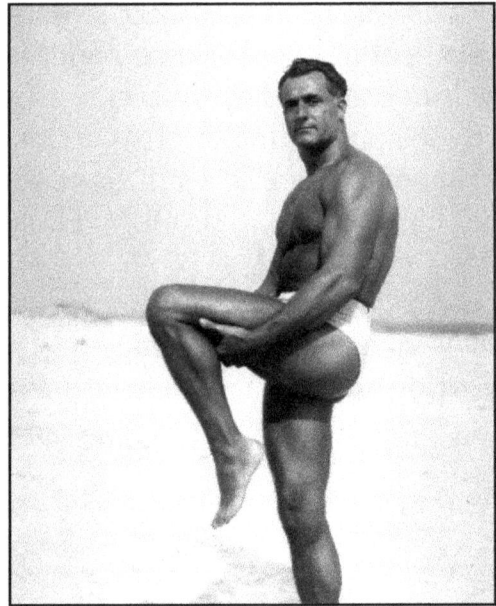

Thigh rows

These are perfect for targeting the upper and lower lat muscles as well as the lower back. Apart from that there's Resisted Across the Body Rows that targets the lats fully from top to bottom. These exercises are under continuous tension within the range of pull. However, with the Thigh Rows resistance drops off a bit at the top position, but by all means a highly effective exercise. Interlock the fingers behind the knee as shown with right leg.

With both arms pull the thigh upwards towards the chest while resisting with the leg. This exercise widens the upper back, works the mid-back and stimulates the biceps as well. Work one side fully then switch to the other side. If balance is an issue perform the exercise seated.

----

05 UPPER-BACK EXERCISES

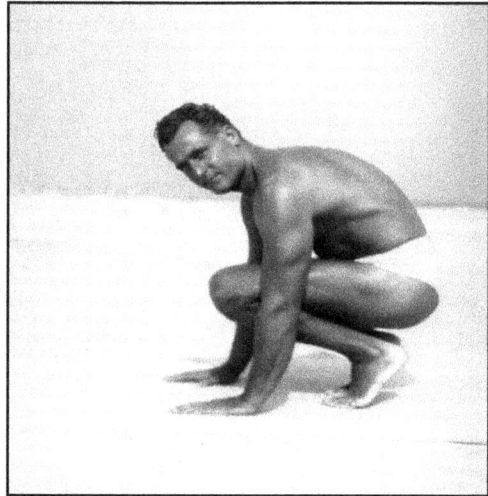

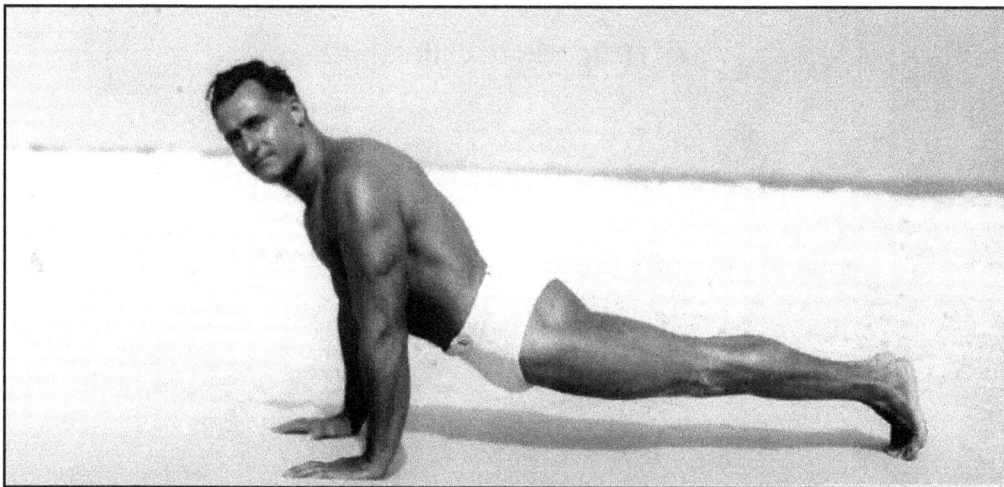

Upper-back kick out

Assume the squatting position above with hands on floor, then, quickly kick the legs out as shown in the pictice above. Then quickly reverse the position to the squatting position. Perform 3 sets of 20 plus reps. This will condition the upper-back as well as conditioning the entire system.

----

05 UPPER-BACK EXERCISES

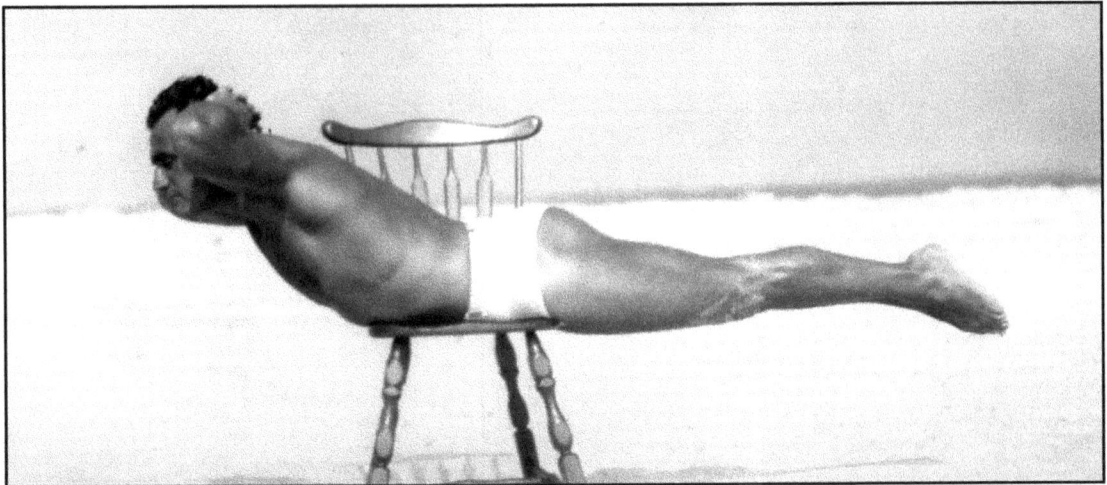

Lower-back extensions

While lying on a chair or stool or simply flat on the floor, raise your upper body upwards until you feel a strong contraction in the lower-back. This is a favorite exercise of mine that stabilize the entire upper-body, plus builds a brace of muscle around the entire spinal structure. Perform 3 sets of 15-25 reps

----

05 UPPER-BACK EXERCISES

Upper-back contraction

Practice this movement at odd moments throughout the day. Pull the shoulders back, grasp hands as in illustrastion and turn slowly but vigorously alternately to left and right. An awesome movement for the upper back muscles.

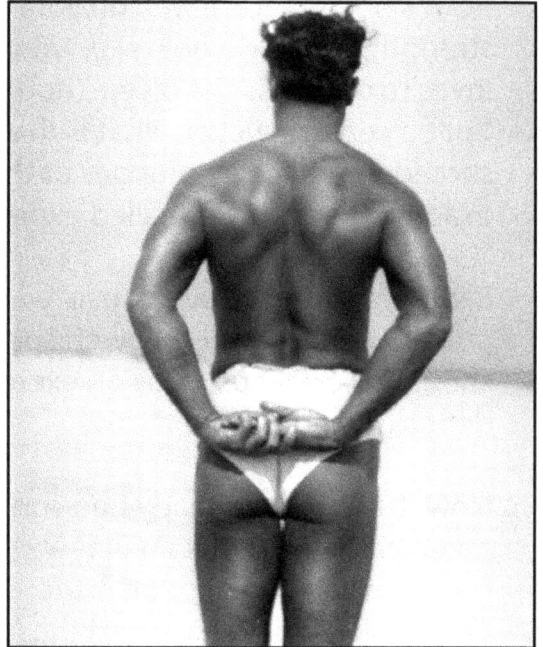

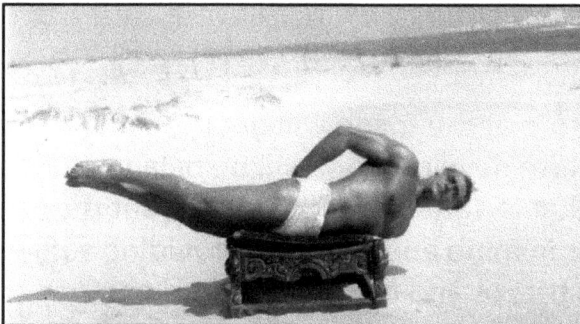

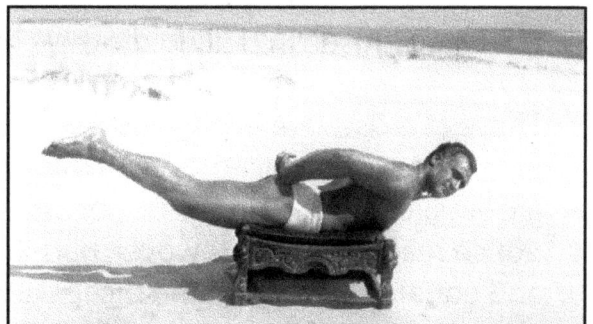

Lower back contraction

In the position above, bend the right side of the body, then assume original position and repeat the movement on the opposite side. Repeat 20 reps at 3 sets per side.

----

06 BICEP/TRICEP EXERCISES

At this point you are well on your way on the road to muscular power and strength. Please do not relax with your training. The very first muscle everyone loves to display is the bicep, (upper arm) because everyone want a pair of strong, built biceps. However, what is the use of an enormous bloated bicep if the shoulders and chest muscles of the chest are not strong and powerful? Yet this is exactly what many so called experts are requesting their students to do!

Earlier within this book consisted of a variety of various exercises for developing a powerful chest, later followed special exercises insuring broad, cannon-ball shoulders. So let us focus on exercises for the upper arm you have something definite to work on.

Now the arm has already had considerable exercise in all the foregoing chapters, and it will be to a certain extent greatly benefited by this preliminary work. Later on when you come to the exercises for developing powerful forearms, and a grip of steel you would have had those exercises to prepare you for that work. In the upper arm there are two IMPORTANT muscle groups, the bicep, to the front; and the tricep, situated at the back. The tricep is used for pushing movements, while the bicep is used in pulling movements.

These exercises are evenly distributed so that the tricep will get the same amount of exercise as the bicep. So, the overall arm development will be balanced. There are smaller muscles in the upper arm, that is right under the biceps but they are not so readily noted. However, bare this in mind and focus on providing sufficient and equal work to both the biceps and triceps and make sure these muscles are receiving their full quota of work.

Before beginning these movements take accurate measurements of the con-tracted bicep with a tape measure, and then observe your monthly improvement. As in all the other exercises you do, practice this wearing just shorts, and perform all your exercises in front of a large mirror. Now, kindly observe this suggestion: Focus on applying enough tension on the muscles being worked however please do not use excessive force!

----

06   BICEP/TRICEP EXERCISES

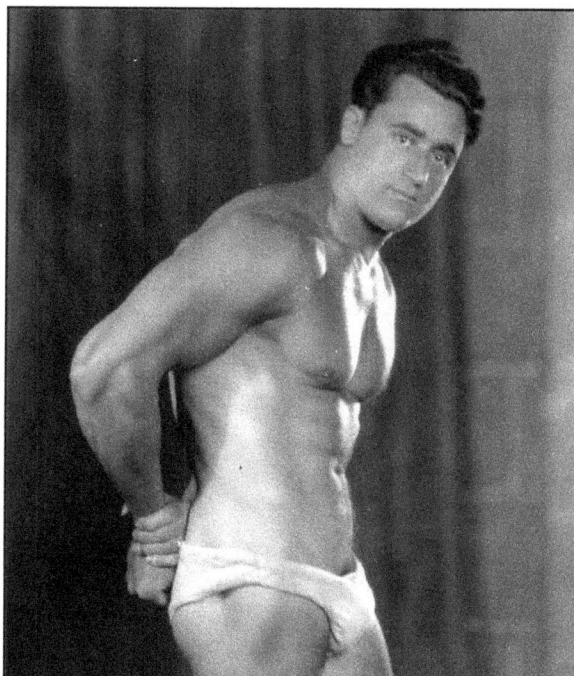

Behind-the-back curls

With your right arm behind your back, place your left hand on the wrist of the right, lean forward until you feel a stretch in the biceps (front of arm). Curl the right arm towards the right arm pit then reverse the movement for 10-15 reps then switch arms.

06 BICEPS/TRICEP EXERCISES

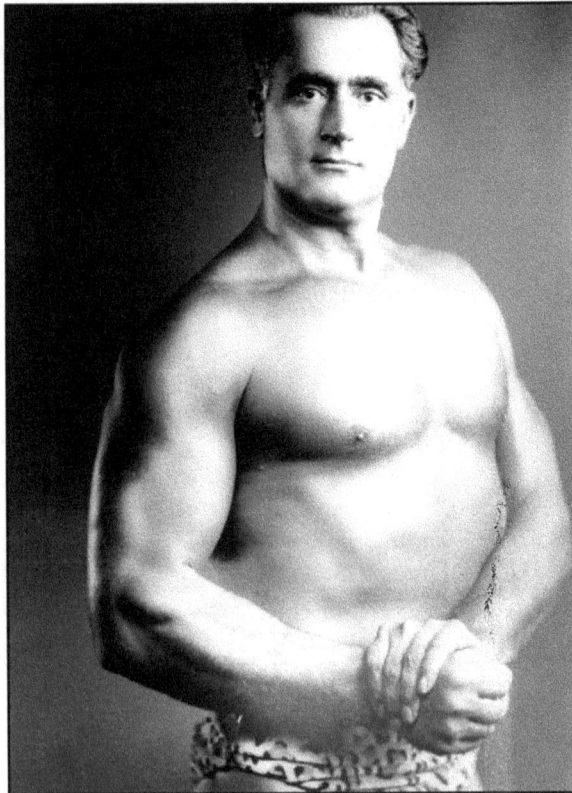

Hammer curls

Another great Bicep/Forearm combo. Place the wrists as shown in the picture above. Now pull with the right hand or bottom hand upwards to the chest while resisting with the top hand. At upper chest level reverse the exercise by pressing the top wrist down and resisting with the bottom wrist. Repeat for reps then switch arms.

06 BICEP/TRICEP EXERCISES

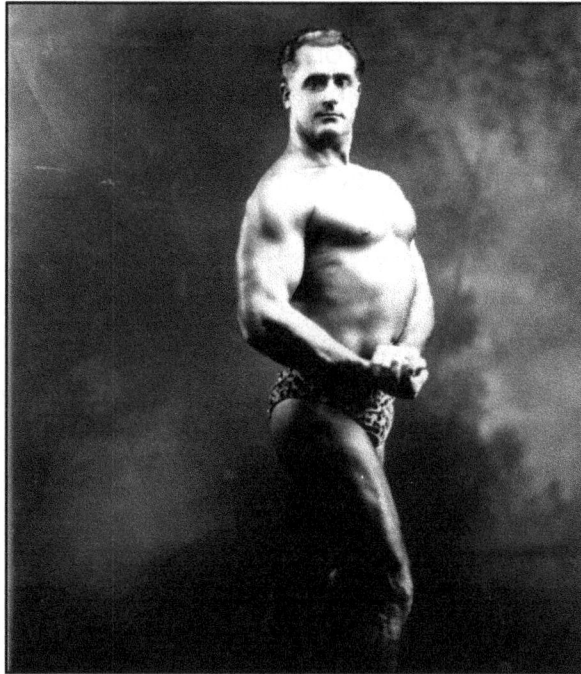

Bicep curls

Grasp your right fist with the left hand. Pull the right arm upward towards the shoulder while resisting with the left hand. At the shoulder, reverse the exercise by pushing the left arm downwards resisting with the right. Continue for reps then switch arms.

---

06 BICEP/TRICEP EXERCISES

You will gain no benefit by going through your exercise plan in a perfunctory manner. Concentrate your attention on their perfection, focus on your exercises. Make this an obligation and keep it in your mind's eye; Focus and DO IT! These powerful exercises will surely build enormous arm muscles once you place plenty of effort into them and carry them out faithfully day by day.

Strength training exercises exhausts the body and nervous system. These exercises tire you for a few moments but gives you increased muscular strength and development. So do not hesitate to put plenty of powerful resistance and energy into each exercise, within doing this the results will begin to show within a few days once you keep at it. You will be extremely surprised at your progress.

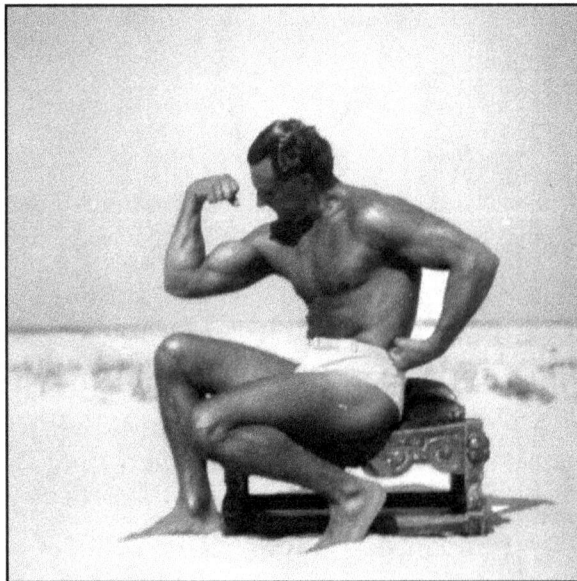

Static contraction movement

This is a static contraction movement, contract the bicep and hold it for 20 seconds three rounds each. Afterwards, be sure to massage the muscles with upward strokes.

---

06 BICEP/TRICEP EXERCISES

However, you will gain no benefit by going through your exercise plan in a perfunctory manner. Concentrate your attention on their perfection, focus on your exercises. Make this an obligation and keep it in your mind's eye; Focus and DO IT! These powerful exercises will surely build enormous arm muscles once you place plenty of effort into them and carry them out faithfully day by day.

Strength training exercises exhausts the body and nervous system. These exercises tire you for a few moments but gives you increased muscular strength and development. So do not hesitate to put plenty of powerful resistance and energy into each exercise, within doing this the results will begin to show within a few days once you keep at it. You will be extremely surprised at your progress.

06   BICEP/TRICEP EXERCISES

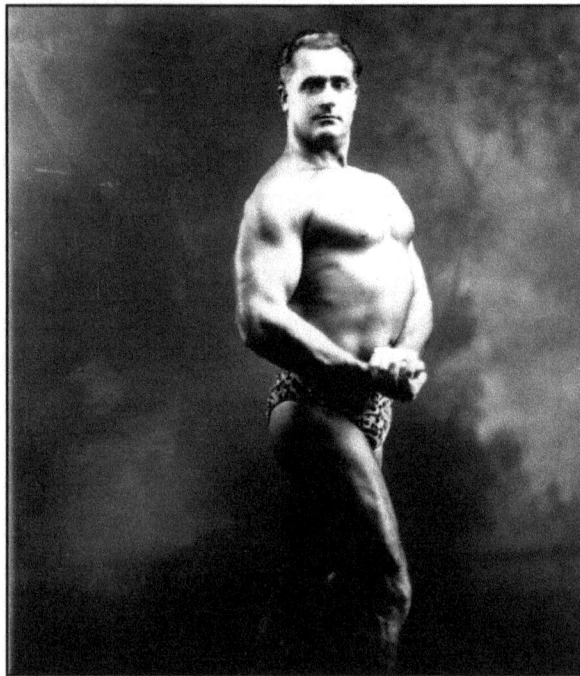

Tricep pressdown

From position shown at right, force right hand downwards while resisting strongly. An ideal exercise for triceps and all the muscles of the upper arm. Work with both your arms, resisting in both directions.

----

06 BICEP/TRICEP EXERCISES

Exercise 1) With this exercise place the right hand against the right shoulder, inter-lock the fingers of both hands and resist with the left while pushing the right arm downwards. A splendid exercise for developing the triceps. Try it with the left arm as well. Continue for 15-20 reps.

Exercise 2) Allow the arm to hang perfectly limp, now vigorously tense the tricep muscle of the upper arm. Compel it to stand out in bold relief. Make it feel hard and solid, by directing the mind into it. Relax, now shake the arm so that it is entirely limp again. While the tricep is tensed, relax the hand muscles. Perform this with one at a time.

---

07 FOREARM EXERCISES

Now, I am giving you the best exercises ever devised for quickly developing powerful forearms. By this time you will have had considerable work for the chest, shoulders and arms to prepare you for these strengthening exercises. After a few week's conscientious practice you will be really amazed at the increased power and endurance you will gain from these simple exercises.
Let's begin.....

Practise shaking your hands with yourself, squeezing and gripping as vigorously as you can with the other hand. Practice this alternately with both hands. Hold the tension for 30 seconds then, reverse hands for the same time time frame.

The above exercises will develop marvelous strength and power of the forearms. However please remember, you can not make any improvement unless you perform the movements faithfully and persistently. Are these exercises simple? You bet they are, but you need to do them and see how vigorous and effective they really are.

At the end of three short months you will develop a steel-like grip, and strong, developed forearms. Do not say you do not have time to do these exercises. You have lots of time during odd moments. A suitable time is upon rising from bed or going to bed. Make the time and utilize these moments, and you will be amazed at the new cords of muscles within the forearms you will develop.

NOTE: A SECRET: Practice them daily, do not miss an exercise session, concentrate on the group of muscles involved, and relax after each set of exercise. Do not strain and overdo the tension. Guard this secret well in your mind for it is the infallible key to your success.

08 THIGH EXERCISES

To maximize development in both your thighs and calves you should walk at least three miles every day. At frequent intervals during the walk, please be sure to force the legs as far backwards and as far forwards as possible. The objective being to give the thigh muscles (and calves) plenty of exercise. Ordinary mild walking is not sufficient to bring out any pronounced muscular development.

The muscles have to be stretched, tensed and fully contracted before any improvement can be made. You see many runners and long distance walkers with more or less thin legs and thighs. Running and walking are excellent exercises because they compel you to be outdoors breathing pure fresh air, but they do not give muscular development as do the properly directed exercises outlined within this book. Therefore, kindly remember to tense the muscles in your thighs and calves at frequent intervals while out walking or running. Make this an everyday exercise without fail.

08 THIGH EXERCISES

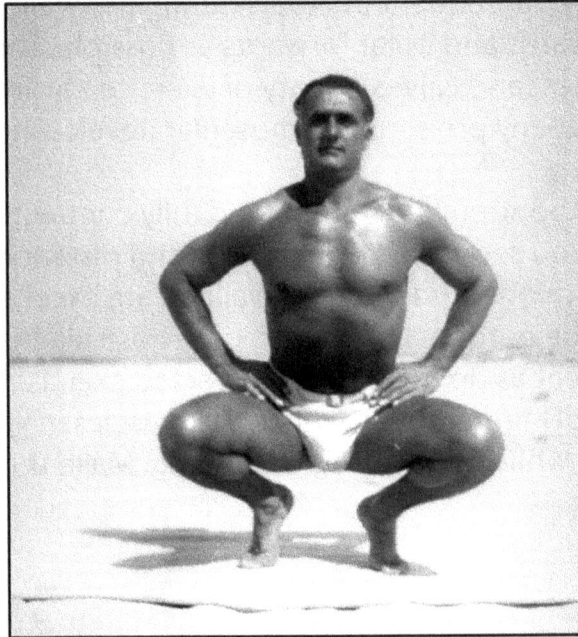

Balance squats

Perform this squatting movement-on the ball of your feet support yourself with your hands lower yourself to the position shown then raise up to the starting position. Fantastic for overall thigh development as well as the calves. To increase and produce greater growth hormone production perform 20-30 reps per set. Once advanced, aim for 100 reps overall for increased development.

08 THIGH EXERCISES

Crossed feet squats

Another excellent exercise for the overall thigh and hamstrings. Start off as shown in the bottom position with feet crossed. Slowly under control push yourself to the finished position. NO BOUNCING! One second pause then reverse the movement to the starting position. This exercise may be difficult at first but keep practicing and as night follows day it gets easier.

Inner thigh flex

Assume the squatting position, sitting on the heels, with the knees wide apart. Grasp the knees with the hands just INSIDE and try to bring the knees together resisting strongly by pushing the hands outward. Continue until tired.

Outter thigh and hip flex

While in the same position as the preceding movements except that the knees are together instead of apart, place the hands on the OUTSIDE of the knees making an effort to spread apart the knees and resisting with the hands. Practice this 20 times for three rounds.

08 HAMSTRING EXERCISES

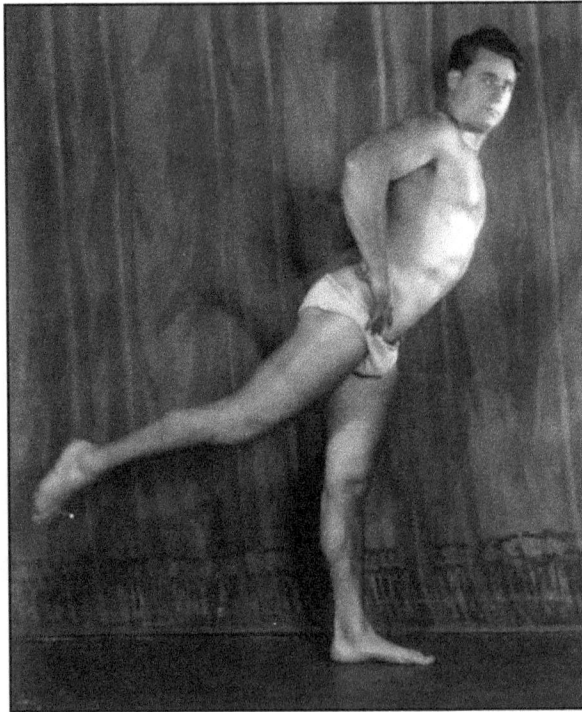

Leg curl

(Hamstrings) For back muscles of the thigh, bend the leg backwards and pull the heel upwards towards the butt, while tensing the muscles of the back of the leg. Practice 20 times for 3 sets each leg.

----

08 HAMSTRING EXERCISES

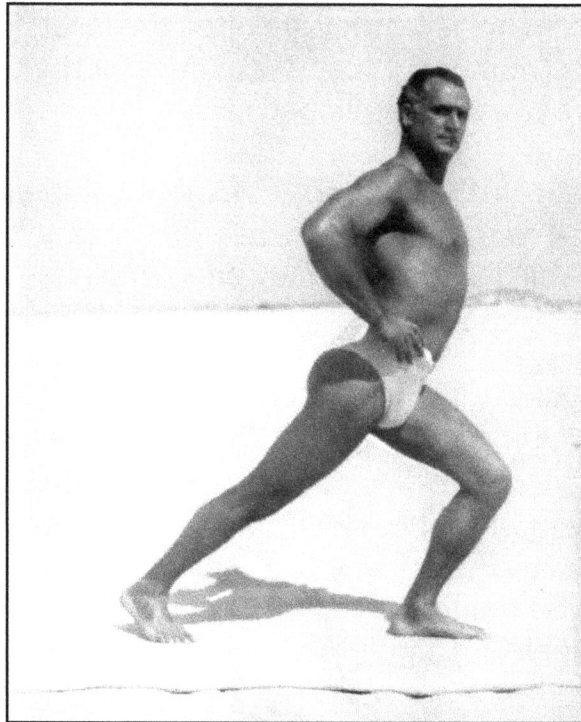

Lunges

(Thighs) As shown, bend left knee, thrust body forward with right foot far backwards. Repeat this "lunge" 20 times each leg at three rounds.

----

09 CALVE EXERCISES

We are almost there! Everyone would like to be proud owners of well developed, diamond shaped calves, however they are often the most neglected of any part of the body. Here are a number of special exercises for the calves, legs and feet in general, they will give you well-developed calves.

The exercises are not at all difficult, and the majority of them can be practiced daily at any moment throughout the day. It is important that you go through all the exercises, as you will discover that they bring into play new muscles you did not realize existed.
Please remember, As a chain is no stronger than its weakest link! So you can not afford to neglect even so-called unimportant muscles.

Performing these exercises will not take very long, and once these exercises are practiced regularly, you will notice steady ongoing improvement. It is a good plan of action to take your calf measurements each month. This will insure that you stay on track with your calve training due to daily perserverence and you will soon be the owner of a great pair of diamond shaped calves.

09 CALVE EXERCISES

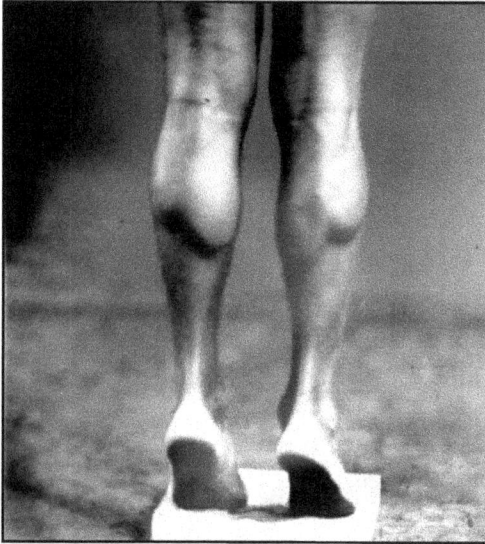

Standing calve raises

On a step rise on your toes as high as possible, tensing the calves vigorously. As you lower the foot to stretch the calf muscles, continue for 25 times at 3 sets morning and night, or if you prefer at odd moments during the day.

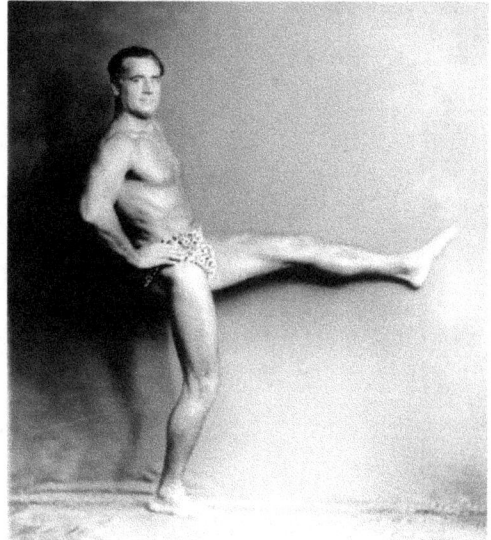

Feet press

Stand on the right leg extend the left foot forward and point the toes forward, then point them towards your upper body. Fantastic for the front part of the shins. Perform 20 reps at 4 sets each foot.

09 CALVE EXERCISES

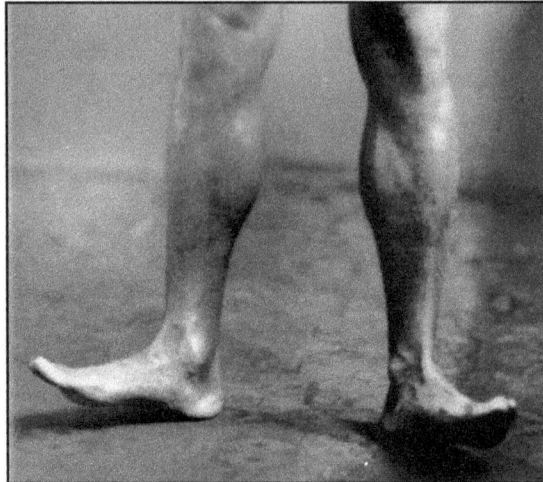

Shin flex

As shown, raise your toes upwards towards your shins tense the muscles, then lower the toes towards the floor. Practise this movement 20-25 times at 3 sets.

----

10 ABDOMINAL EXERCISES

Strong abs, everyone wants them. A slender stomach, a powerful mid-section, It is equally important to have strong powerful arms and a iron cord forearms, but of what use are these unless the abdominal area is in perfect condition?
Why not keep this power-packed system working effeciently with added strength. This will be accomplished by a proper systematic exercise plan.

The exercises suggested within this chapter are very simple, but at the same time extremely powerful and effective. You will start seeing results day by day, both in increased radient health and internal muscular power and strength you will gain from these exercises. The abdominal muscles will stand out firmly like wash board abs. So, let's get cracking!

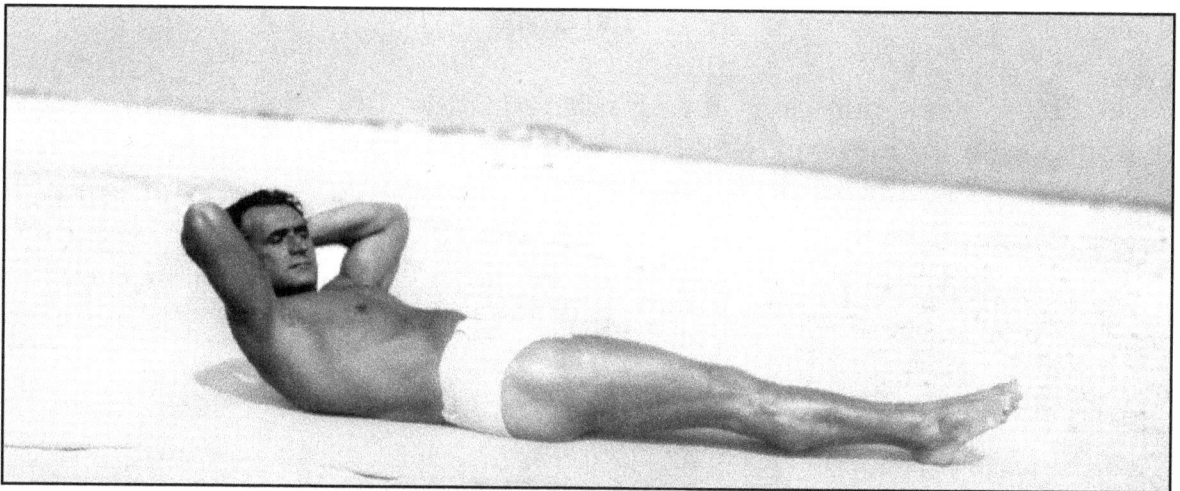

Full range sit-ups

While lying on your back, raise your upper body forward bringing the head over so that it touches your knees. Not only do you achieve powerful abs you will gain massive flexibility within your hamstrings. Perform 20-25 reps at 3 sets daily.

----

10 ABDOMINAL EXERCISES

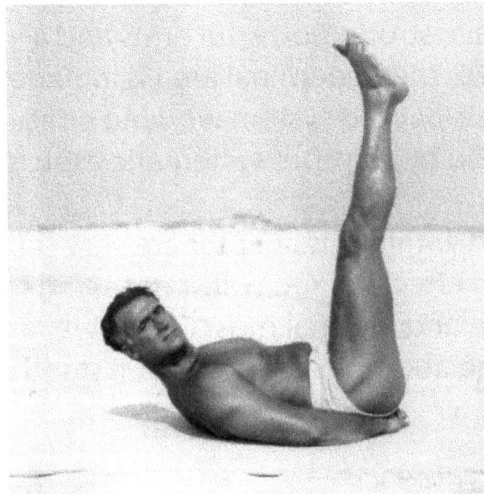

Leg raises

As shown, place your hands at your sides and raise your legs towards your upper-body. Lower the legs and repeat. Perform 20 reps at 3 sets daily.

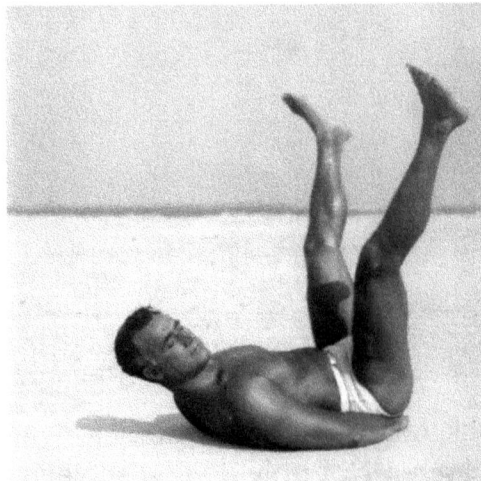

Lie on your back, raise feet, spread them out as far as possible. Now cross the legs in an X position alternating the legs. Perform 25 reps at 3 sets.

10 ABDOMINAL EXERCISES

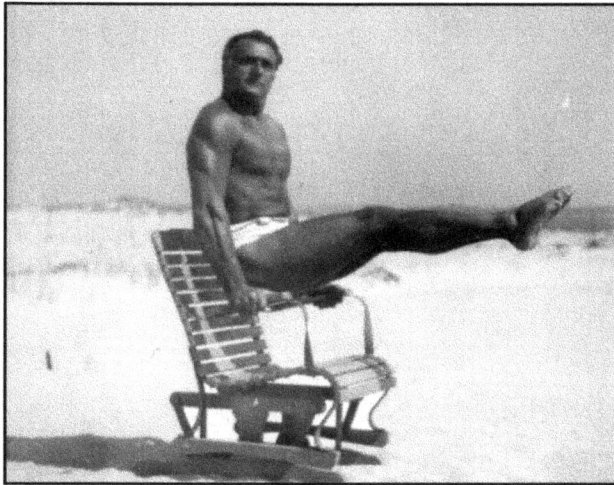

Chair dips

Grasp hands firmly on arms of a chair. Bring feet to position shown, bend your elbows and lower your body. Then reverse the motion by pressing back up. This is a difficult exercise, but a little practice will enable you to do it many times. As you gain muscular power in your abs and triceps.

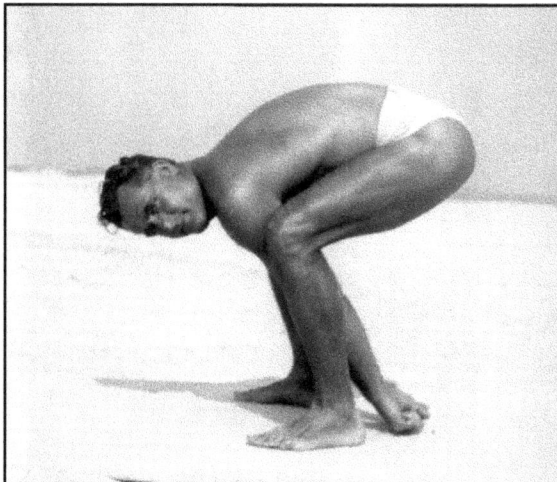

Stand with feet 20 inches apart. Bend knees and lower body. Extend arms between legs and touch floor. Reach as far back as possible, tensing your abdominals. Continue forcing hands further backward, keep the abs tight. Perform 20 reps at a time for 3 sets in total.

10 ABDOMINAL EXERCISES

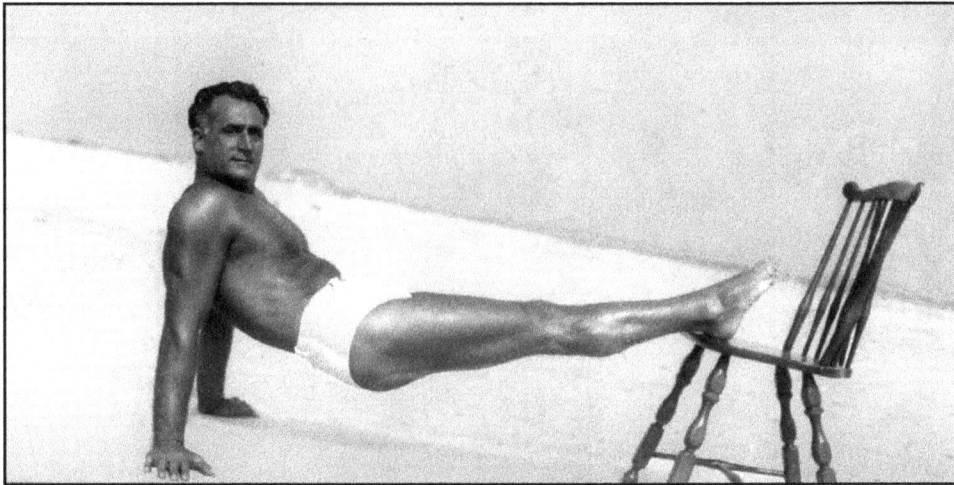

Reverse decline dips

From position shown, bend the elbows and permit the upper-back to touch the floor, then press the body to original position the level of the chair. A very effective for the abs and upper body.

----

11 MASTERING THE TRUE TONIC OF LIFE

CONQUERING WORRY AND ANGER

My experience in dealing with human nature is that I have found few people who were not inclined to worry and anger at some time of their lives. While it is a recognized human weakness, fortunately it can be helped. Worry, irritability and anger are mental and physical poisons. By giving vent to these undesirable habits the body tears down far more quickly than it can be built up. I suggest that you do not worry or get very angry. However, occasions may arise when you will have a fit of anger and it is well to know how to throw off the mood.

It is known that babies have been killed by poisoned milk from angry nursing mothers. This illustrates the terrible consequences of anger and worry on the physical body. On NO account allow yourself to become worried, either over the past, the present or future. The past is dead. Forget it! Why dig up the corpse? The future has not arrived, why anticipate what probably will never happen? Plus, why worry over the present? Will your worry accomplish anything positive?

Will it benefit you any? It will not. Then why worry? Cut worrying out of your life forever. Allow yourself to live on the sunny side of life. Companions with large souls, think pleasant thoughts. Worrying is a nasty habit that drains one's vitality; they are a waste of one's time and mental energy. They poison the blood and prevent the best and quickest development of a perfect body. It is proven: Worry works its irreparable injury through certain cells of the brain, and that delicate mechanism being the nutritive center of the body, the other organs becomes gradually affected in a negative way.

Worry and fear retard not only the brain but the functioning of the entire digestive system. Thus if you eat while worried, you can expect a good case of indigestion. Don't fret. Force yourself to relax and get out of that mood. Try to laugh, even think of the funniest things you can recall that happened to you. Every morning of each day read some inspiring thoughts, and focus on this throughout the day. This will keep you in a positive mindset.

----

11 MASTERING THE TRUE TONIC OF LIFE

CONQUERING WORRY AND ANGER

In other words, substitute your worry-some thoughts and reverse it for thoughts of health, strength, happiness and joy. Enjoy life, get all the sweetness and happiness out of life as you can. Make the best of your life in every respect. It is your right to be happy. Train your mind and your body WILL follow! This will indeed have a powerful effect on your physical body, giving it added power and magnetic charm. Saturate your life with plans of the future, positive, constructive ideas and ambitions and there will be no time, or desire to worry.

The following suggestions are given by a well-known philosopher, and you are urged to scorch them deep into your soul: ELIMINATE FEAR, CONQUER WORRY, AVOID ANGER, OMIT DEPRESSION, SHUN HATE, STUDY CHEERFULNESS, CULTIVATE HOPE, DEVELOP COURAGE, EXHIBIT CONFIDENCE, ASSUME SUCCESS, LIVE SIMPLY, CONTROL SELF, CULTIVATE HAPPINESS, FOCUS ON HEALTH YOURS, plus CULTIVATE HAPPINESS.

Do all you can to make yourself and others happy. This will soon reflect itself in your life. For remember, health and happiness go hand in hand. CONTINUE THIS REGIME UNTIL YOU ARE THE MASTER. FOCUS ON THE VALUE OF AIR AND BEING OUTSIDE IN THE SUNSHINE AS A HEALTH AND STRENGTH BUILDER.
Charles Atlas advised all students to take their exercises as far as possible in just shorts and in front of a large mirror, the reason? For motivation, while seeing your muscles pumped with blood and seeing the muscles contract.

The skin need to breathe and if covered by clothing it has little chance to get the air it needs. The sense of freedom without clothes alows the skin to breathe, Charles Atlas called this air baths. Whenever possible your air baths should be taken while basking in the warm sunshine, but be ever so mindfull to apply sunscreen for added protection.
These combined air and sun baths can be taken anywhere lying in the garden, in the bedroom or other convenient places where the sun can shine through the open window. If you can get out into the country and enjoy these baths it is even

----

11 MASTERING THE TRUE TONIC OF LIFE

CONQUERING WORRY AND ANGER

The morning is a good time to take these sun and air baths, but of course be careful not to get burnt. The sun's rays on the body have the same influence as on plants and flowers. If you hide a beautiful flower in a dark cupboard you know that flower will soon wilt, fade and die, but when placed in the warm sunshine it soon blooms in all its magnificent glory.

The same applies to your body. There is life and vitality in the rays of the sun, which seekers of bodily perfection will not miss getting. Then again, the air and sun have a soothing influence on the nerves, calming and quieting them in a natural manner. If the air is pure and cool it is a splendid tonic to the skin and entire body, and has often proven a good method of preventing colds.

The ultraviolet rays of the sun impart vitamin D to your body. Pure air and the sun's warm infrared and ultraviolet rays are the best germicides and most powerful disinfectants we have.

----

12 AQUIRING PHYSICAL MAGNETISM

At this point you would have been more than satisfied with the results already secured by using these self-resistance methods. In the previous chapters you have been instructed in how to exercise every muscle group for maximum muscular development. Now that we are at the final stages of this course, do not neglect the methods outlined for you. You have acquired the habit of exercising daily – please keep it up.

SPECIAL METHODS FOR ACQUIRING PHYSICAL MAGNETISM OF SPECIAL IMPORTANCE

As of today avoid every habit which you know to be injurious to your health, or practices which will not promote the best physical condition. This is especially important in regards with diet, drink, sex and tobacco in excess.

Each morning, take a cool shower to cool off the body followed by muscle-stretching and deep breathing. Take this shower immediately upon arising, and you will feel a warm glow over the entire body after the bath. During this operation throw the magnetic WILL into it and every effort connected therewith.

Two or three times each week vigorously massage your scalp making it move with your fingers. Massage carefully every part of the head and conclude the magnetic stimulation by massaging gently.

At least once each day the facial muscles should be pulled into all sorts of contortions, massaged with clean hands, and exercised completely by voluntary movements. This keeps away wrinkles and flabbycheeks, giving the face a pleasing appearance and expression. Plus, maintain daily scrupulous cleanliness of the hands, feet and teeth.

In the evening the feet should receive a tepid bath with a cool rinsing especially during the warm weather. This strengthens the feet and ankles, keeping them in good condition at all times, and prevents that tired feeling so many experience after their regular day's work. Each and every day throughout life practice full deep abdominal breathing, empty the lungs as much as possible, disregard the chest, and depress the diaphragm by muscular effort, pushing out the abdomen.

----

12 AQUIRING PHYSICAL MAGNETISM

Now slowly fill the LOWER lungs, slowly exhale, relax and repeat several times. Again empty the lungs, disregard the abdomen and swell out the chest with muscular effort, slowly filling the upper lungs. Slowly exhale, rest and then repeat a few more times. Now while standing erect, lungs empty, swell out the chest and abdomen, pushing down the diaphragm, slowly filling the lungs as much as possible. Relax and repeat, see that the air is fresh and cool. Also practice these exercises while walking.

During each experience throw the will into each inhalation, ordinarily the breathing should be ABDOMINAL, by pushing the diaphragm downwards. Remember, the body cannot live for more than a few moments without oxygen, and the larger volume of air - within reason - you take into your lungs the healthier and stronger the lungs will become.

In addition to the deep breathing exercises occasionally perform the following muscle-stretching and relaxing exercises. When stretching see that the movements are slow and gradually increased in intensity to their utmost limits. Likewise the relaxing must be gradual from stiffness to complete limpness.

As muscles you exercise are becoming stiff fill the lungs full of pure air. During the period of relaxing, slowly empty the lungs. Avoid jerky movements, but see that they are gradual with the mind concentrated intensely upon the muscles involved, saying to yourself: I am now increasing my muscular strength and magnetism!.

The first part of the body you are required to stretch is the neck. Stretch the neck far backward while inhaling, slowly exhale while relaxing and allow the head to slowly fall far forward quite limp. Concentrate the mind on the neck. Vigorously stretch the right shoulder and inhale deeply, then relax slowly. Alternate the method by using the other shoulder. Repeat a few times.

----

12 AQUIRING PHYSICAL MAGNETISM

Stretch out the right arm as far as it will go, make a further effort to reach out still more. Inhale at the same time. Relax. Repeat with the other arm. This movement will include stretching the forearm, upper arm, wrist and fingers. Now stretch the chest outward and upward as far as it will go while taking a full deep breath, gradually relax. Repeat twenty times.

While sitting, bend the back at the upper part slightly forward. Stretch it as much as possible, pushing out the elbows at each side, making a fanlike shape of the upper back. Relax and repeat a few times. When out walking stretch powerfully the rear foot, pointing the toe backwards a second. Stretch the whole thigh, leg, calf, ankle, the foot and toes. Make it as vigorous as you can without straining.

As the other foot is in the rear stretch that, relaxing as you bring the foot forward in the usual course of walking. While these are simple exercises they become dynamic as you direct the WILL into each movement, giving each movement definite concentrated attention. These special exercises are not to be confused with the regular exercises for developing physical perfection which you are to take in the morning and at night.

The special movements indicated above are to be taken during the day at odd times, while out walking or waiting. They form excellent supplementary exercises to the regular ones. Under no circumstances continue these movements beyond the fatigue point. If you persist in going beyond that point you tear down the muscular tissue, doing more harm than good. To get the best and quickest results perform vigorously all motions with a WILL, continue the movements until SLIGHTLY fatigued - THEN STOP and relax.

The value of these special magnetic exercises is achieved by the stretching and combined deep breathing. This draws increased supply of rich pure blood to the parts focused on,this creates large quantities of oxygen, and thereby builds up the tissues making the entire body a Power-House of Energy.

12 AQUIRING PHYSICAL MAGNETISM

The total length of time in performing these simple but effective movements is but a few moments, and there is no excuse for not going through them regularly each day. While an ox may have perfect health, it is not magnetic.
The subtle quality you wish to acquire is like that of an Arabian steed, which is both powerful, healthy, virile and MAGNETIC.

Simple laws of nature, performed in the spirit of HOPEFULNESS combined with this compelling power of radiant health is the result of obedience to the DIRECTED WILL. You may increase this POWER by carrying out the instructions in this course with alert, energetic and EXPECTANT ATTITUDES, which you should endeavor to make permanent in your life.

The benefits of these simple but powerful methods if persistently followed will enrich your life and bring you splendid health, prosperity and happiness. Keep up the instructions as far as possible throughout life. If you care to send me your photograph within the next few weeks showing the results accomplished, I shall be glad to receive it.

Your next and final chapter I call the Perpetual Lesson. In it are the best Isotonic Tension exercises for you to do daily to keep in perfect shape.

----

13 PERPETUAL DAILY PRACTICE PROGRAM

To get the maximum benefits and most extrordinary results from my Course some of the exercises should be carried out faithfully throughout life. You have developed the habit of exercising regularly and on a daily basis to achieve ultimate results. However, for Life-Long Health and Strength do the following exercises daily. They are what I believe you need most to keep you fit **LIFELONG.**

EXERCISE NO.1
For Chest, Shoulders and Triceps. Excellent for preventing Lung and Chest troubles. Perform the incline pushup exercise as described in the first chapter at least 100 times every day. Aim for 200 times daily if you are keen on getting a very powerful chest development. Perform 20-25 times, at 3 sets. If you prefer, perform 50 to 75 at night. Charles Atlas performed 200 incline pushups daily.

EXERCISE NO. 2
For the Abdomen. Ideal for reducing a large stomach. While lying on the floor clasp the hands back of the head and raise the upper body so that your chin touches your knees, keeping your feet flat on the floor. Perform 20-25 times. Rest awhile and repeat for 3 sets.

EXERCISE NO. 3
While in the same position, perform a leg raise. This should be done until you are thoroughly tired, perform 20-25 reps at 3 sets. Another variation for this movement would be to open and cross the legs but only for variation.

EXERCISE NO. 4
For Thighs. Perform the squatting exercise spreading apart the knees. Repeat at least 35-50 reps at 3 sets. Perform this exercise energetically. Rest and repeat as before, now for taxing the inner thighs and hamstrings keep the ankles close together.

This will develop and stress the muscles of the back of the thighs. If balance is an issue, rest one of your hands on something for support. These exercises can be performed in the morning as soon as you get up or before getting ready for work.

13 PERPETUAL DAILY PRACTICE PROGRAM

EXERCISE No. 5

Developing Biceps, Triceps, Arms and Forearms. Grasp the right wrist with the left hand in front and bring the right hand towards the right shoulder, resisting powerfully with the left hand. Pull up and press the arm downwards with the other arm in a dual manner. Resisting in both directions. Perform 15-25 reps, continue till the muscles really begin to ache. Then repeat with the other arm. Rest and do them again for 3 sets each side. This exercise can also be done with the right palm faced downwards as you curl upwards.

EXERCISE No. 6

Strengthening your neck. Bend the neck far downwards, then far backwards. Also, from side to side, resisting in both directions. Rest and relax. Perform these exercises with moderate tension by powerfully resisting with the hands. These are very effective exercises once done persistently.

EXERCISE NO.7

To build the back part of the shoulders and upper back muscles. Across the body pulls are a great choice. Place your arm across your chest with the right arm, now place the left hand on the right elbow. Now, pull the right arm towards the right hip resisting with the left hand. Perform 20 reps at 3 sets each side. Resist in one direction only.

EXERCISE NO.8

Add massive muscle and strength to the upper and lower back muscles. Thigh rows, perform this exercise by bending over and grasp with both hands under the thigh, just behind the knee. Now pull the thigh upwards with both arms towards the chest. Resist in the up motion only while resisting with the leg, perform 15-20 reps at 3 sets each side.

EXERCISE No. 9

Calves, Perform this exercise on stairs or a block where you can stretch the foot downwards to add lenth to the calve muscles. Another good exercise is to stand on the heels and rock back and forth first on the heels and then on the toes. Do this till really tired. Rest a few minutes and repeat as before. These exercises can be performed at night, just before getting into bed. Some of them, however, can be done at odd moments during the day.

13 PERPETUAL DAILY PRACTICE PROGRAM

EXERCISE No. 9

Calves, Perform this exercise on stairs or a block where you can stretch the foot downwards to add lenth to the calve muscles, perform 25 reps at 3 sets. Another good exercise is to stand on the heels and rock back and forth first on the heels and then on the toes. Do this till really tired. Rest a few minutes and repeat as before. These exercises can be performed at night, just before getting into bed. Some of them, however, can be done at odd moments during the day.

When out walking make a practice of stretching the entire legs and calves to the full limit. Be sure and raise up your toes as you walk along. By keeping this up for a distance equal to ten blocks you will soon have a fine pair of well-shaped legs. These exercises may seem like a long routine to practice daily for the balance of your life but, thousands upon thousands of men are doing them daily, and very busy men, too, so do not say you have no time.

You will find when you divide the exercise, doing half in the morning and the other half at night it takes only a few minutes. In closing, it has been a pleasure and I truly enjoyed putting this course together, for I know you must be Stronger, Healthier, more Muscular and full of Energy. It has been a pleasure to help you. Men and women like you will live longer and enjoy life more.

Please tell your friends about this course so they can enroll, so that I can help them, gain powerful muscles in double quick time too. Although this chapter completes my Course. Hope you are enjoying the newly found muscles all over your body.

----

14   fEATS OF STRENGTH IMPORTANT!

Do not expect to do these feats of strength the very first time you try them. A little practice is required in order to make sure that you do not strain or hurt yourself.

NO. 1 - TEARING A THICK TELEPHONE BOOK

Grasp the telephone book with both hands and bend it over one knee. Slant the pages at the same time so that when you begin to tear you are actually tearing only one page at a time. After tearing all the pages then grasp each half across your chest and tear apart. Use the same idea in tearing a deck of cards.

NO. 2 - BENDING A SIXTY PENNY- WEIGHT NAIL

Wrap a handkerchief very fully around each end of the nail, making sure that the ends do not protrude and injure your hands. Grasp one end in each hand keeping them close to your chest and then start to bend the nail with your hands pushing with your shoulders at the same time. After you have bent the nail a little more than half way, interlock your fingers of both hands putting the nail in the center and squeeze it so that it is completely bent making the ends touch. In this trick speed is of great importance. Once you start bending the nail you should continue to bend it.

NO. 3- DRIVING A 3 1/2 INCH NAIL INTO TWO PIECES OF 1 INCH PINE WOOD

Place a 1 inch thick piece of wood across the back of two chairs so that when you drivethe nail through the wood it will not damage anything. Then, wrap a cloth such, as a large handkerchief, carefully around the head of the nail so that it wont hurt the palm of your hand during the blow. Holding the nail point down give it a hard blow straight down on the wood. If the head of the nail is carefully wrapped you will find that you can give a real heavy drive without feeling any of the shock in your hand. The nail should come out through the wood perfectly straight. At first try a 1 inch piece of wood then the two pieces.

NO. 4- BENDING A STEEL BAR 5 OR 6 FEET LONG AND 1/2 INCH THICK

Take a raw steel bar and place a piece of cloth around the center. Then put the bar in your mouth and hold tightly with your back teeth around the cloth. Balance the bar with your arms and have one light weight man on each side pull downwards on the bar. Be sure to balance the bar so as to avoid injury to your jaw. In this manner you will be merely balancing the bar and the men will be actually bending the bar. Be very careful not to damage your teeth.

----

14 fEATS OF STRENGTH IMPORTANT!

NO. 5 - PULLING AN AUTOMOBILE WITH YOUR NECK

Put a leather strap around your neck and attach to rope which is tied to the front axle of the car. Then slowly pull backwards while facing the car, making sure that the strap around the back of your neck will not slip. By tensing your back, shoulder and neck muscles, you will be amazed how easily you can pull a car.

NO. 6 - LIFTING A CAR BY THE REAR BUMPER

This trick is performed by grasping the rear bumper while your back is towards the car. Start with your knees bent and then straighten up. The rear of a car is much easier to lift, due to the fact that the motor is in the front while comparatively very little weight is in the rear of the car.

NO. 7 - LIFTING A MAN HEAVIER THAN YOURSELF

Facing the man grasp his right bicep with your left hand, place your right hand inside of his right thigh. Then have him lean towards you in a rigid position and then lift him up, straightening your elbow as you lift. If this trick is done correctly it is very easy to lift a man of considerable weight. It is important that the man you are lifting keeps his body rigid.

NO. 8 - ONE HAND LIFT

Standing in back of a man, place your right hand in the middle of his lower back. Both of his hands are to be on your wrist and with your left hand holding his left ankle. The man is to give a jump upwards and backwards and you are to straighten your arm, and at the same time straighten your legs. Thus with your arm straight overhead, the man will actually be sitting on your hand.

NO. 8 - ONE HAND LIFT

Standing in back of a man, place your right hand in the middle of his lower back. Both of his hands are to be on your wrist and with your left hand holding his left ankle. The man is to give a jump upwards and backwards and you are to straighten your arm, and at the same time straighten your legs. Thus with your arm straight overhead, the man will actually be sitting on your hand.

----

14 fEATS OF STRENGTH IMPORTANT!

NO. 9 - LIFTING A PONY

Place a good harness, that will not slip, around the stomach of the pony. Attach a loop on the harness on one side of the pony. With your back to the pony place your right arm through the loop and you will be amazed to find how easily you can lift the pony on your back.

NO. 10 - HOLDING TWO CARS EACH GOING IN THE OPPOSITE DIRECTIONS

Attach a leather strap to the rear of two small cars. Arrange the cars with the backs to each other. Then stand between them with one on each side of you. Attach the leather straps from the cars to your arms. Interlock your hands and get a good footing. Then have the cars slowly start together in opposite directions. By keeping your hands tightly interlocked the cars will actually be pulling against each other and you will apparently be holding back both of them. Great care must be exercised lest you hurt yourself by the cars starting too fast, or by one starting too soon.

CONCLUSION

Before attempting to perform these feats you should be sure of your strength and accuracy in handling these tricks. Also be careful not to over-exert or strain yourself.

----

14 fEATS OF STRENGTH IMPORTANT!

HAND BALANCING

When one is learning a hand-stand it is necessary to have some sort of support in order to give the beginner confidence in himself. It is therefore advisable to begin by doing the handstand against the wall. Stay about two feet away from the wall. Put your hands flat on the floor, fingers spread apart, put all your weight forward and be sure to keep your elbows firm, and head up.

Kick up with your feet resting them against the wall and arch your back. When you have held this position for a few seconds bring your feet away from the wall.

The secret of the hand-stand is to keep your arms straight, your back arched and head up. Also keep the toes pointed legs together. Follow the above instructions carefully and practice this everyday, I am confident you will be able to do a perfect hand-stand within a month.

When practicing if you lose your balance fall to the side or to where you started from. Do NOT fall backwards as there may be a danger of hurting yourself.

When you are able to hold a perfect hand-stand for about ten seconds, try to dip down and up again. This is a marvelous exercise for both arms, shoulders and chest, also for the internal organs such as kidneys, stomach, etc. It relieves the strain on the muscles that hold the internal organs such as the stomach, bowels and liver. It is also very good for poor circulation.

When you become very sure of the two arm hand-stand so that you can stand on your hands as well as your feet you can try the one arm hand-stand. This is done by putting all your weight on one side holding the hand that is free out sidewards. The legs in the one arm hand-stand are spread apart so as to make balancing easier. Do not be discouraged if you not successful the first few times you try these, but remember that perseverance is the key to success.